Homemade Healing Salves

30 Recipes of Balms and Ointments for Different Kinds of Injuries

Table of Contents

Introduction

For different kinds of health issues, there exists various solutions and using the natural herbs and other natural ingredients is the best way to get rid of dangerous infections. Getting your injuries and wounds treated by the natural remedies is an amazing way of using the natural resources for the benefit of mankind.

The book includes 30 excellent recipes of balms and ointments for treating various kinds of wounds and injuries. All the ingredients included in these recipes are very suitable for your usage and doesn't provide any side effect. They are all easily available and very easy to be used in crushed forms.

You can store these creams and balms for long time and can use whenever you get any bruise or cut. This would save your body from get fatal infections.

Chapter 1 – Natural Remedies for Wounds and Injuries

Nowadays, plants are the main source of different strong drugs for various modern plagues such as cancer and heart diseases. However, there is an amazing variety of the homemade herbal remedies used in the field of medical. Before going in detail of making of these remedies, it is important to know the essential benefits of the main ingredients used in these remedies.

Following are the few herbal ingredients with their amazing benefits:

1. **Eucalyptus oil:**

    The pungent smell of the oil of eucalyptus (which is usually called as the fever tree) can get through however your nose is stuffy. Spread some drops of the oil on a piece of cloth and then breathe in vapors of oil, or spread some of the oil on the pillow before you go to sleep.

2. **Catarrh cure:**

    The collection of the sweetly scented stimulant and antibacterial herbs can be utilized in form of chest rub (after being diluted with the neutral oil like olive oil and almond oil) or can be inhaled, for making the breathing easier.

3. **Lemon and honey cough linctus:**

    There are the two cold remedies after the third one – whisky – so this can be used only by adults, which serve best for the treatment of cough.

4. **Red sage sore throat gargle:**

    This is a great homemade remedy for the sore throat and is very powerful than the other remedies.

5. **Ginger:**

Ginger is used for nausea including travel and morning sickness, even pilots take it with them during flights.

6. Chamomile tea:

This is known as the mother of gut because of its healing characteristics. It relives stress and insomnia.

Chapter 2 – Top 15 Ointment Recipes

Usually it is the common concept of the people that it is very difficult to make the herbal ointments because there is a matter of calculation and accurate measurement of all the ingredients. On the contrary, the experience of many people and experts has shown that it is the easiest and the simplest task to formulate the herbal medicines and ointments. Herbal ointments are simple to make. The biggest advantage of making these medicines at home is that you can reduce the cost of medicine per jar to considerable amounts. Particularly the specialty stores sell these ointments and medicines for much more prices than their actual costs of making. Another great advantage of these medicines is that you can not only make them at hand for yourself but these also make very good and useful gifts. A few recipes with easy to find and cheap ingredients are as follows:

1.   Healing salve:

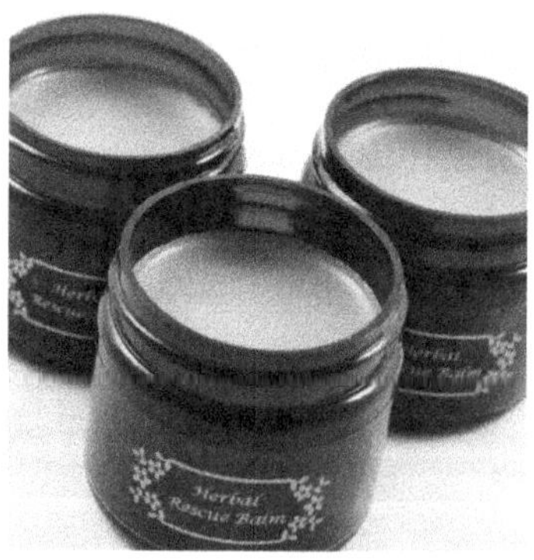

Ingredients:

For making this ointment you need to have following supplies:

> ➢ Ovenproof dish

> ➢ Double boiler
> ➢ Cheesecloth or a mesh strainer with fine mesh
> ➢ 1 cup of olive oil or any other carrier oil of your choice
> ➢ 1 cup of the herb of your own choice
> ➢ ¼th cup of beeswax
> ➢ A dry and clean jar for storing your ointment

Directions:

First of all, start your oven and heat it up to 200°. After heating it to the desired temperature, turn it off. Now put the oil along with the herbs in a double boiler. The purpose of boiler is to heat the mixture and not completely boil it. For this purpose, keep the boiler on a medium heat. You only need to heat the mixture until the mixture reaches at a steep heating point and it does not boil. After the oil mixture is heated to considerable value, and then you need to stick the top most part of the boiler to oven for a few hours.

After you keep the boiler in oven for a considerable time period, you need to remove the herbs from the solution. For this purpose, you can use the cheesecloth or a steel wire mesh. It totally depends on you if you want only the oil with herb extracts of you want the herbs infused in it for some more time. Now put the oil again on the burner on a medium heat. Now add beeswax in this oil and stir until all of it as melted. Finally pour this mixture in the jar and save it for use.

2. *Wound healing ointment with antibacterial properties:*

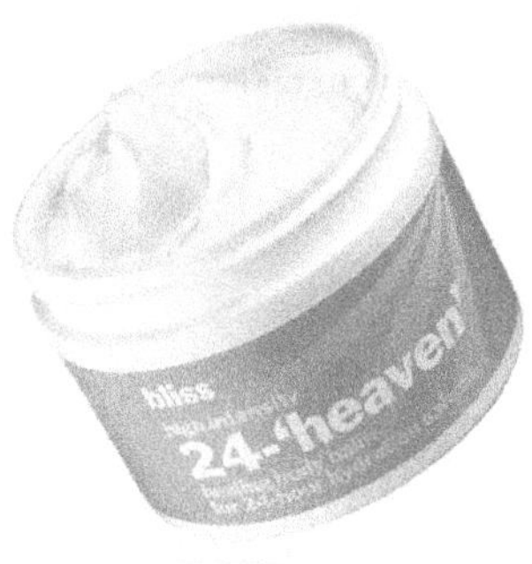

Ingredients:

- ➢ 2 Tbsp. of coconut oil in refined form
- ➢ 2 drops of the tea tree essential oil or the oregano essential oil
- ➢ 2 drops of the essential oil of helichrysum
- ➢ 2 drops of the essential oil of lavender
- ➢ 2 drops of the essential oil of frankincense
- ➢ 1-2 tsp of the pastilles of beeswax. However, this ingredient is optional.
- ➢ 1 ounce of salve tin

Directions:

First of all, melt the coconut oil in a double boiler. Basically there is a need to melt it. In addition to this if you are also using the beeswax, then melt it along with the coconut oil the oil in winters. After the oil is liquefied, there is no need to heat it further. Instead start adding the essentials oils one by one. Add the essential oils one at a time and not simultaneously.

Now mix all the oils together and then pour the mixture in a jar or a small tin. Now you need to put the mixture in fridge to let it cool down and solidify. This ointment is excellent to be applied on minor cuts and scrapes. If needed, you can then apply the bandage as well.

3. *Ointment to be applied on the burns and wounds:*

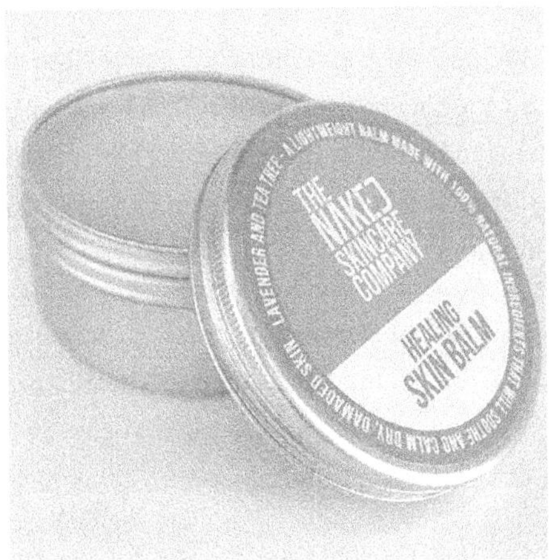

Ingredients:

- ➢ Dried comfrey, root of marshmallow, warm wood and bark of witch hazel 1/4th ounce each.
- ➢ 1 1/4th cup of olive oil or any other oil according to your choice
- ➢ 4 ounces of raw honey
- ➢ 1-2 ounces of beeswax

Directions:

First of all, weight al the dried herbs on the kitchen scale. In the next step you have to prepare the infusion of these herbs in oil. There are three ways of making the oil infusion of herbs. These procedures are listed below:

Cold infusion method:

In this method take the weighed herbs in the jar of glass mason and cover the herbs with the olive oil. Then stir the mixture to combine and coat the herbs with oil completely. Now this mixture is let steep for about 4 to 6 weeks.

Hot oil extraction method:

Take a glass mason jar and cover the herbs with oil in the jar. Stir well to combine the herbs and oil. Now place the glass jar on a cook pot so that it is filled with water and keep the heat of stove on the lowest setting. Infuse the mixture of herbs and oil on stove for about 4 to 8 hours for one day or for up to 3 days. Keep an eye on the pot and add more water when it evaporates continually.

Now strain the mixture on a cheesecloth and squeeze out most of the extract from the mixture. You must make sure to extract maximum of the oil from the mixture. Now take a saucepan and melt beeswax on a very low heat. The quantity of beeswax depends on the thickness of your slave which you want. Now add this to the oil mixture and mix it completely. Allow it to cool so that it begins to harden. At this stage stir the mixture in a blender until a creamy and smooth mixture is obtained.

4.   *Ointment cream to be used as first aid:*

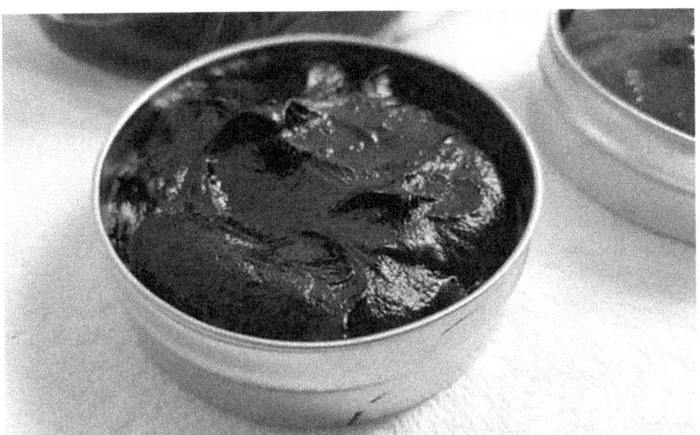

Ingredients which you require for ointment making:

> ➢ 250 grams of either petroleum jelly or soft paraffin wax
> ➢ 30 grams of the dried herbs of your own choice

Directions:

Take a bowl and place it over a pan of boiling water. Melt the petroleum jelly or paraffin wax in this bowl. You can also melt it in a double saucepan. Now add the herbs in this molten jelly or wax and heat the mixture gently in the pan for about two hours. After heating it for two hours, pour the jelly mixture in a jelly bag or on a piece of muslin cloth which is already fitted on the edge of a jug. Secure it with the piece of rubber string so that it may not droop down with the weight of jelly mixture. Now wear rubber gloves before handling the jelly mixture because it is still hot. Squeeze the mixture in the jelly bag or muslin cloth. After that transfer it in the jelly jars while it is still warm because once it is solidified, it will be difficult to transfer it in jars and you will have to heat it again. Do not secure the containers with lid until the mixture has cooled down completely because otherwise it will result in making of crystals.

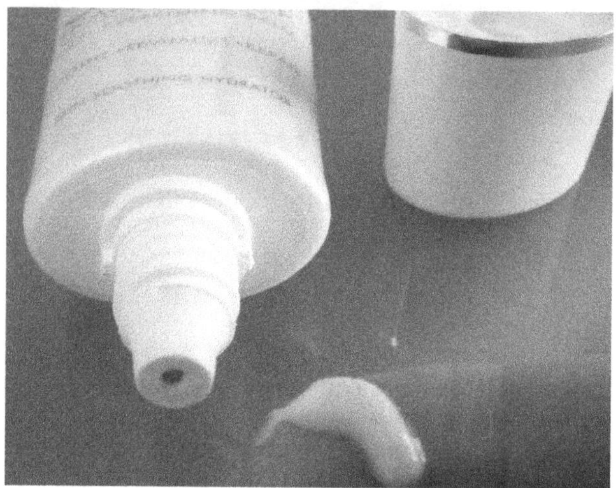

Ingredients for making the cream:

- ➢ 1/2 cup of coconut oil
- ➢ 2 teaspoons of the pellets of beeswax
- ➢ 2 teaspoons of the camphor crystals or 5 drops of camphor oil
- ➢ 2 teaspoons of the menthol crystals or 5 drops of peppermint oil in case you do not find the crystals
- ➢ 5 drops of the eucalyptus oil

Directions to prepare the cream

First of all, melt the solid ingredients, which are the coconut oil and the beeswax together in a container. You can melt these in the microwave oven or in a double jar as well. Some people also melt these ingredients directly in a saucepan on a stove for one or two minutes. You really do not mean to heat them up; instead you need to melt them only. After mixing the mixture, allow it to cool and then add camphor crystals or camphor oil in it. After that add menthol crystals or oil and eucalyptus oil one after the other. After stirring the mixture thoroughly, put the container to cool down completely so that it changes its texture from liquid to solid.

When you will apply this sold cream on your akin, it will liquefy again and will absorb into your skin. This is the perfect property of the creams which are used for massaging on the sprains, sores and injured muscles and joints.

6. *Ointment made from coconut oil and garlic for skin treatment:*

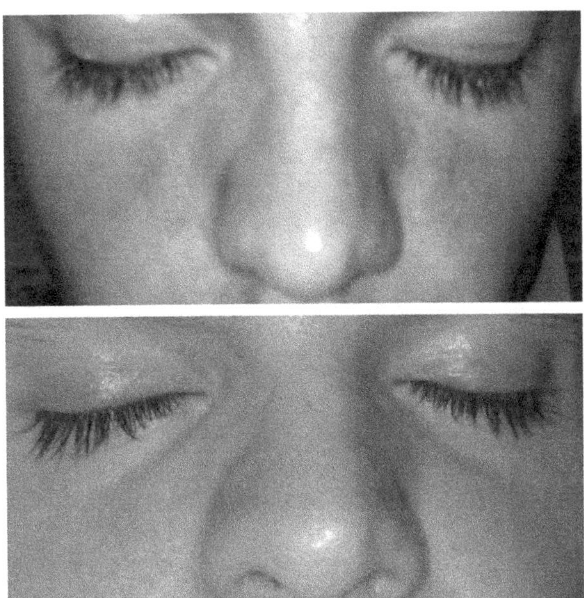

This ointment is very useful and it soothes the dried skin thereby healing it from deep inside and also nourishes it. Basically it will also help your skin to regain its moisture and lost nutrients.

Ingredients:

- ➤ Unrefined coconut oil 3 tablespoons
- ➤ Extra virgin oil 3 tablespoons. The extra virgin olive oil has enhanced properties because it is treated by cold press treatment.
- ➤ Garlic crushed and chopped, 1 teaspoon
- ➤ Jar with wide mouth and a lid

Preparation of the ointment:

First of all, warm out the coconut oil in a pan so that it melts. Now add an equal quantity of olive oil in it and mix thoroughly so that the two oils mix together completely. After mixing the two oils remove the mixture from pan and add garlic in it. Now pour this mixture in a blender and blend well to get a finally uniform mixture. Strain this mixture so that any solid chunks of garlic, left behind are removed which may have been missed as a result of blending. Now pour this mixture in a jar with wide open mouth and let it cool. It is advised to keep this ointment refrigerated.

7. *Magical anti-wrinkle homemade cream:*

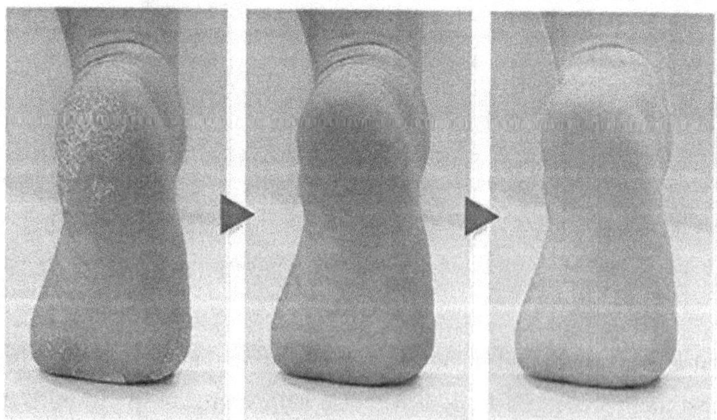

Ingredients:

- 1 1/2 ounces of almond oil
- 1 ounce of Calendula oil which makes about 20 ml
- 3/4 ounces of beeswax or 20 grams
- Dried calendula flowers for infusion
- 1/2 teaspoon of the essential oil of frankincense
- 1/4 teaspoon or 1 ml of the lemon essential oil

Method of preparation of cream:

Make an herbal infusion with the help of the calendula flowers and boiling water. You can make this herbal infusion by placing the flowers in a jug and then adding boiling water form over them. Then leave the jug covered and let it cool down. Now melt the beeswax in a large pan with heavy base. Add to this molten beeswax, sweet almonds while go on beating it by means of a wooden spoon or a whisk. Now add 2 tablespoons of the infusion in the form of a slow trickle.

Now remove the saucepan from stove and keep on stirring so that the cream cools down to almost the body temperature. Now at this temperature add the essential oils as mentioned in the ingredients list according to the measured quantities. After adding the oils stir them completely. Stir till the cream cools down so that the water and oil does not separate from each other. Now spoon this cooled mixture of cream into the jars and make sure that the jars are preserved well.

8.   Recipe of black slave:

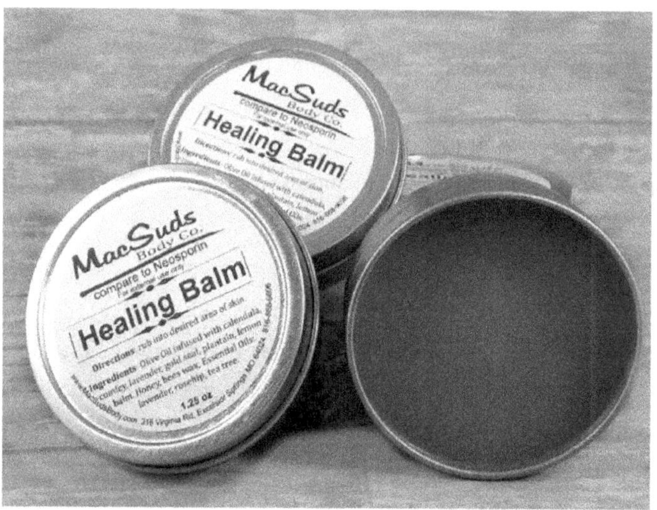

Ingredients required to make the mix:

- ➤ 3 tablespoons of olive oil infused with calendula, plantain and comfrey
- ➤ Shea butter 2 teaspoons
- ➤ Coconut oil 2 tablespoons
- ➤ Beeswax 2 tablespoons
- ➤ Oil of Vitamin E 1 teaspoon
- ➤ Activated charcoal powder 2 tablespoons
- ➤ Kaolin clay 2 tablespoons
- ➤ Honey 1 tablespoon
- ➤ Lavender essential oil in drops

Instructions for making black slave:

The first step before starting the preparations of slave is to infuse the olive oil with herbal flowers. In this cream you have to infuse the olive oil with flowers of comfrey, calendula and plantain. For this you have to take 1 tablespoon of each herb in finely powdered form and mix it in half cup of olive oil. You can mix well the whole ingredients in a blender or mixer.

If you want to make the infusion by cold treatment method, you have to mix the herbs in olive oil and let them stand in it for 3 to 4 weeks. Shake them daily and then strain after 4 weeks by the help of cheesecloth. Now it is ready for use.

Another way is to prepare the infusion in a double boiler. Simply heat the herbs in oil on a double boiler. Leave the heat on medium setting for about an hour. After that the color and smell of the oil will change and it will give a strong fragrance. Finally strain the mixture using cheesecloth and the oil is ready for use.

9.   *Cream for skin care during summers:*

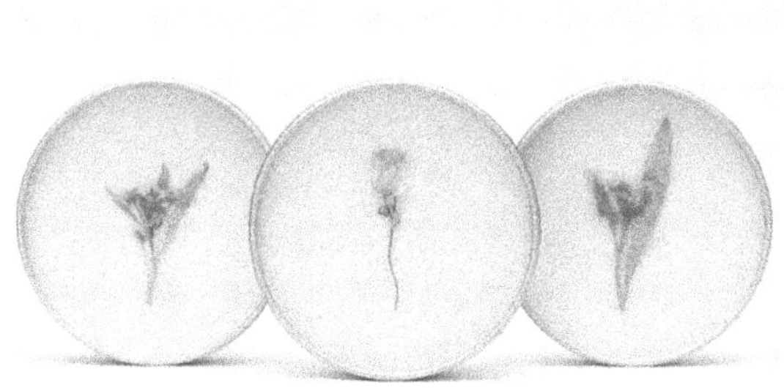

Ingredients required for making the cream:

- ➤ 4 ounces of dry herb or 6 ounces of wilted herb
- ➤ 8 ounces of olive oil or any other carrier oil

Method of preparation of the cream:

In order to prepare the cream, place the ingredients in pan on a stove. Heat the mixture so that it reaches the temperature of 90 to 100 degrees. Now warm the mixture gently after lowering down its temperature. This should be done for about 2 to 6 hours. You can switch on and off the heat periodically. The herbs may not be cooed nor should the oil be smoked. Instead keep the heat under control to maximum extent. After the heating procedure is completed, strain the mixture on cheesecloth or a clean muslin cloths so that a clear solution is obtained. This cream can be stored in a glass bottle and can be used up to 12 months.

10. *Arnica Ointment:*

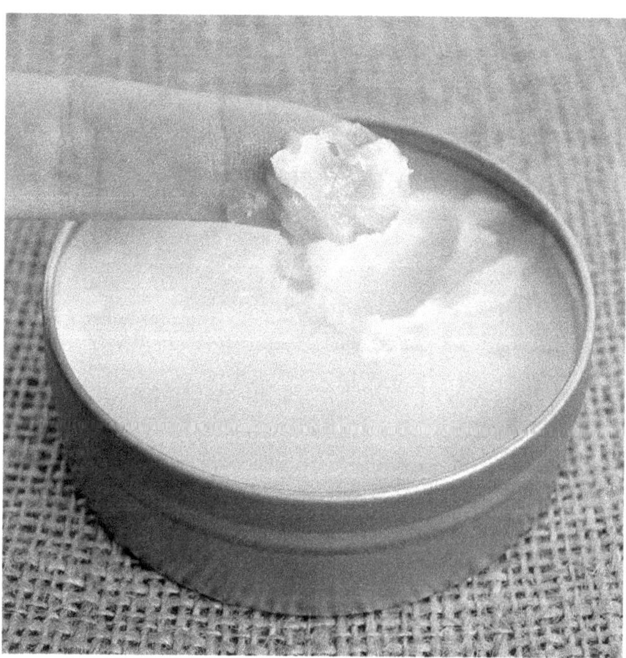

Ingredients for the making of ointment:

- ➢ 20 grams of beeswax
- ➢ 25 grams of coconut oil
- ➢ 20 grams of shea butter
- ➢ 3/4ᵗʰ cup of arnica
- ➢ Infused oil
- ➢ 2/3ʳᵈ cup of helichrysum hydrosol

Directions for making the ointment:

First of all, begin the making of ointment by melting the shea butter, beeswax and coconut oil together in a pan. After melting the mixture completely and homogenizing it, add the infused oil and stir thoroughly on a double boiler. While you pour the oil, you will see that the beeswax will start to solidify again. Therefore, you have to stir everything very well so that all the mixture has the uniform composition. If necessary, gently heat the mixture to melt all the ingredients. When the ointment turns to solid, make sure that it is not too hard otherwise it will become difficult to set the cream.

11. *Recipe of the original capsaicin cream:*

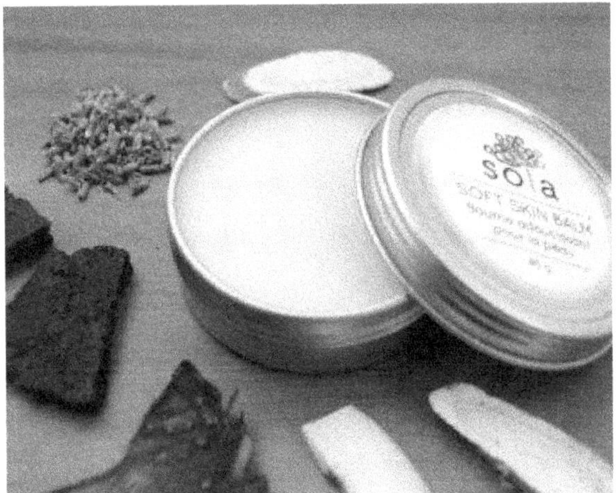

Ingredients:

- ➢ Cayenne powder 3 tablespoons
- ➢ Grapeseed oil 1 cup
- ➢ Grated beeswax half a cup
- ➢ Double boiler for heating the ingredients
- ➢ Airtight glass jar with a lid for storing the cream

Directions for making the cream:

Take the cayenne powder and mix it in 1 cup of oil of your choice. Heat the oil in a double boiler for about 5 to 10 minutes by keeping the flame medium. Now add half cup of grated beeswax and keep on stirring the mixture so that it blends completely. Now chill the mixture and put it finally in the glass jar. You can also whip it again before putting in the jar.

12. *Super-Strength Cream:*

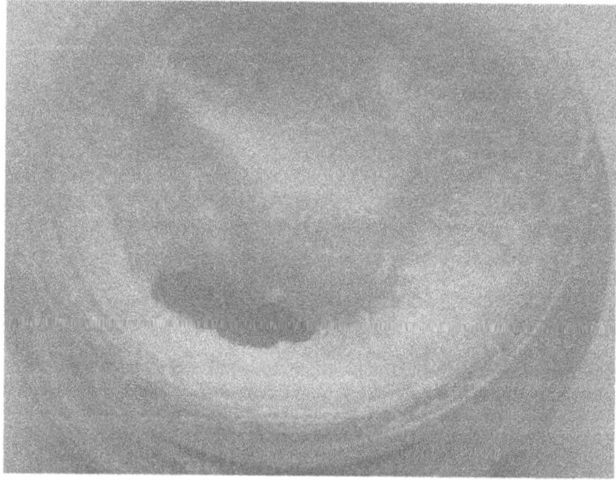

Ingredients:

- ➢ Beeswax
- ➢ grapeseed
- ➢ Habanero powder

Directions:

Mix habanero powder with grapeseed in boiler. Heat it for 10 minutes and then add melted beeswax in it. Stir it and chill for 10 minutes.

13.   *Healing Cream:*

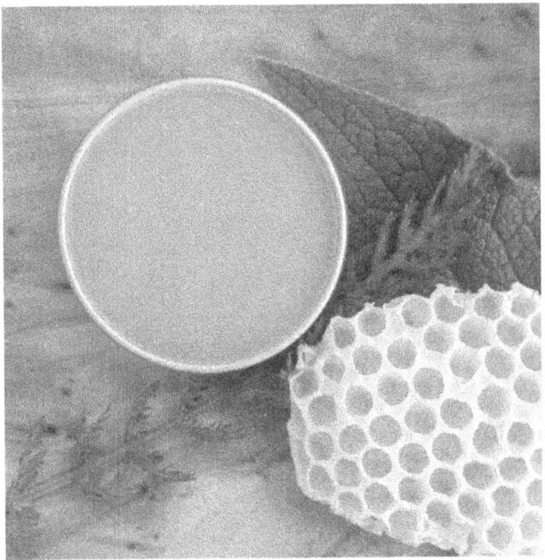

Ingredients:

- ➢ Beeswax
- ➢ Grapeseed oil
- ➢ Turmeric
- ➢ Ginger
- ➢ cayenne

Directions:

Mix cayenne, turmeric and ginger together. Add grapeseed oil in the boiler and stir. Warm for 10 minutes and add beeswax. Stir well and chill for 10 minutes.

14.   *Burn ointment*

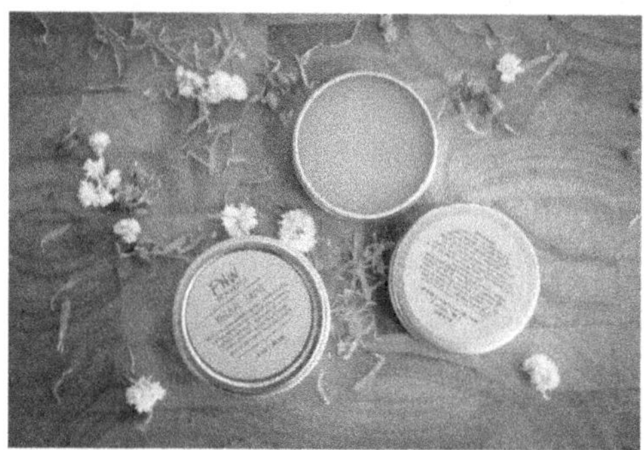

Ingredients:

- ➤ Calendula flowers
- ➤ Comfrey roots
- ➤ Beeswax
- ➤ St. John's Wort flowers
- ➤ Olive oil

Directions:

Add calendula flowers, comfrey roots, and ST. John's wort flowers in a boiler with olive oil and boil it. Let it simmer for 60 minutes and strain it. Add beeswax and heat at low.

15.   *Rub for sore muscles:*

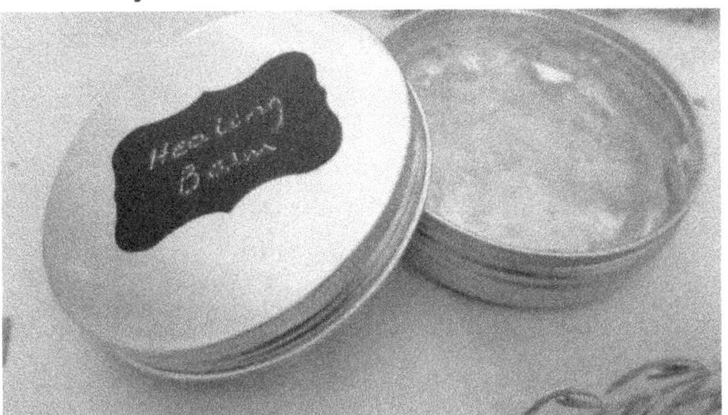

Ingredients:

- ➢ Coconut oil
- ➢ Olive oil
- ➢ Beeswax
- ➢ Clove oil
- ➢ Eucalyptus oil
- ➢ Ginger
- ➢ Peppermint oil

Directions:

Add coconut oil, olive oil in pan with ginger and pepper. Heat in water for 20 minutes. After this add beeswax and heat till it melts. Put the mixture in strainer and add peppermint and eucalyptus oil. Both providing soothing effect to muscles.

Chapter 3 – Top 15 Balm Recipes

16. Strawberry flavored lip balm recipe:

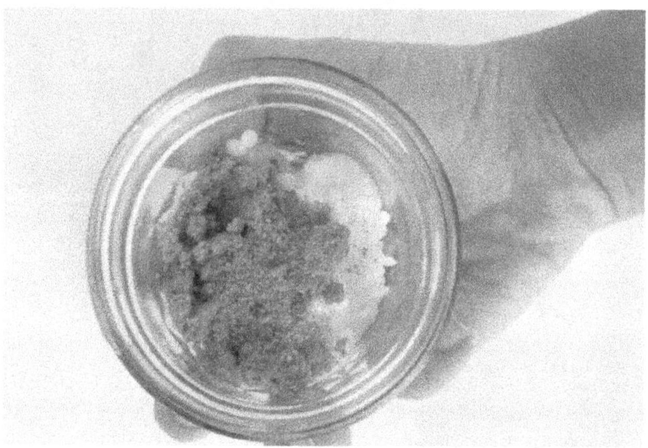

Ingredients:

- ➢ Half tablespoon of sweeten almond oil.
- ➢ Half tablespoon of coconut oil.
- ➢ Quarter cup of frozen strawberries.
- ➢ 1/8 tablespoon of oil containing vitamin E.
- ➢ One tablespoon of pastilles beeswax.

Directions:

1. First of all, grind dried, frozen strawberries in a blender till they are converted into fine particles.
2. Use glass or plastic Mason jar to store all the ingredients from heat and moisture.

3. Now put that jar into boiling water. In such a way that water does not enter into the jar. Water should cover half outside of the jar.

4. While water bubbles are forming, mix it continuously with a chopstick, metallic spoon or with Popsicle stick till completely liquefied.

5. Empty mixture into final the vessel after passing through a strainer. Spare seeds and mash will remain in the strainer.

6. Keep the mixture in a cool place. Stir it after every ten minutes so that color and flavor spread equally.

7. Your lip balm is ready to use now.

17. *Bread and shear butter balm recipe:*

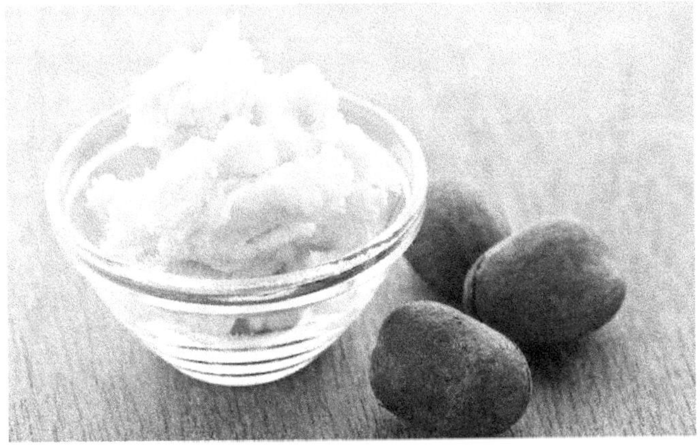

Ingredients:

- ➤ One tablespoon Aloe Vera gel
- ➤ Few drops of lemon grass oil
- ➤ Two drops of lavender oil
- ➤ Curved salve tin
- ➤ Food processor

> Two tablespoon of shear butter
> Cedar wood oil

Directions:

1. Merge all the ingredients and displace them into salve tin.
2. Place it in refrigerator for half an hour until it solidifies.
3. Now it is ready to use. Put some amount on your palms and gently apply it on you beard. After applying sometime can wash it.
4. Sooner you will see an effective change with moisturized and dressed beard.

18. Beeswax Home produced lip balm:

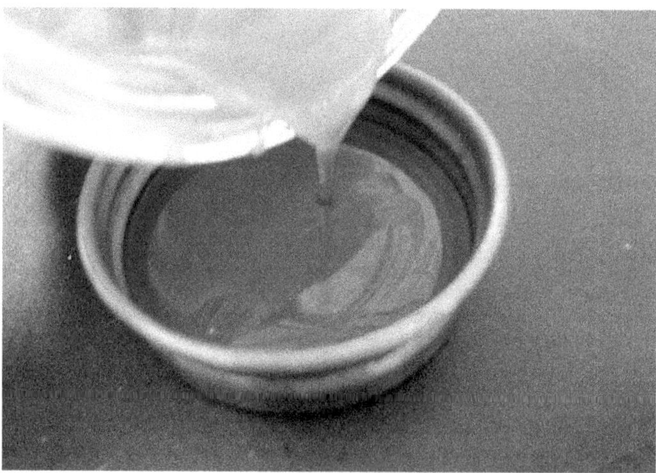

Ingredients:

> One tablespoon of raw honey.
> One tablespoon of coconut oil.
> Few drops of peppermint oil.
> Three drops of rosemary oil.

> Around ten lip balm tubes or pots.
> Some vitamin E oil.
> One tablespoon of grated butter.
> Two tablespoons of beeswax pastilles.

Directions:

1. Use Mason jar and add measured an amount of coconut oil, butter, and beeswax.
2. Take sauce a pan, put the jar in it and fill one and a half inch of water. Heat water to bubbling. Mix it till mixture is liquefied. Note: water must not enter into the jar.
3. Remove it from flame and gently add vitamin E, oils and honey with continuous stirring.
4. Let it settle down and then pour them into lip balm pots or tubes.

19. *Muscle soothing homemade balm:*

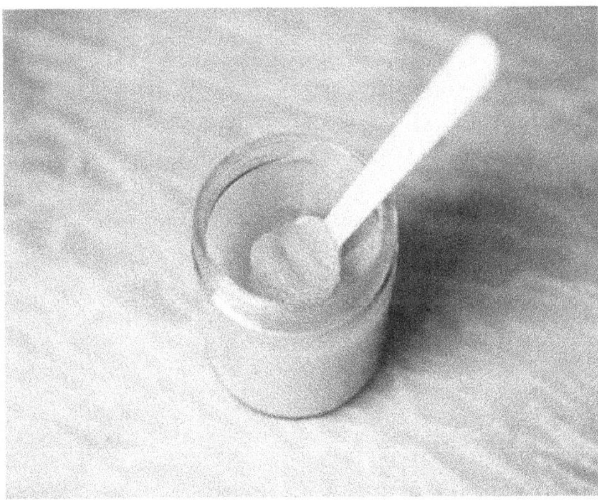

Ingredients:

- ➤ Fifteen drops of peppermint oil.
- ➤ Equal drops of lavender oil.
- ➤ Half cup of coconut oil.
- ➤ Two tablespoons of ginger or turmeric powder.
- ➤ ¼ cup of grated beeswax.
- ➤ Two teaspoons of cayenne powder.
- ➤ A glass jar.

Directions:

1. Add coconut oil into a glass jar.
2. Put a jar into a sauce pan filled with two inches of water.
3. Stir add ginger/turmeric powder and cayenne. Allow contents to melt.
4. If ingredients are properly merged, then add peppermint and lavender oil.
5. Mix it. Finally, pour mixture into a storage jar and allow to set.

20. Face aging skin balm:

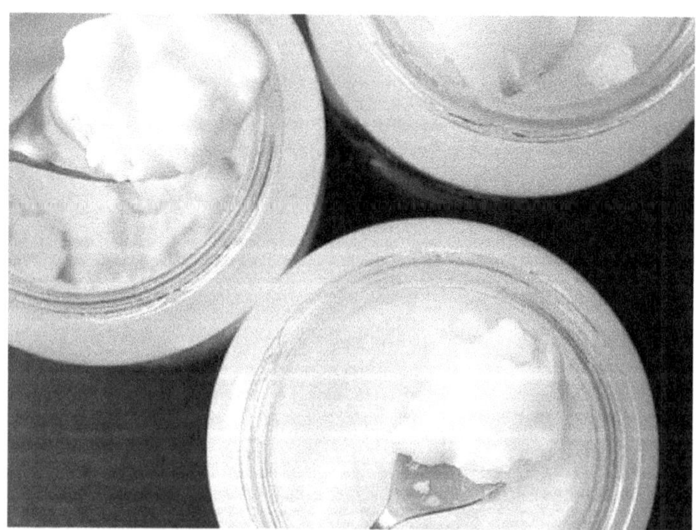

Ingredients:

> ➢ Two drops of helichrysum oil.
> ➢ Six drops of organic frankincense oil.
> ➢ Two drops of lavender oil.
> ➢ Half oz of rosehip seeds oil.
> ➢ A container with dropper and half oz dark bottle.

Directions:

1. Pour all the ingredients into half oz dark glass bottle via dropper.
2. Mix them all through rolling bottle between hands.
3. You can apply it after cleansing your face.
4. You can store it for a long period only if kept in the dark and cool place.

21. *Homemade Eczema balm:*

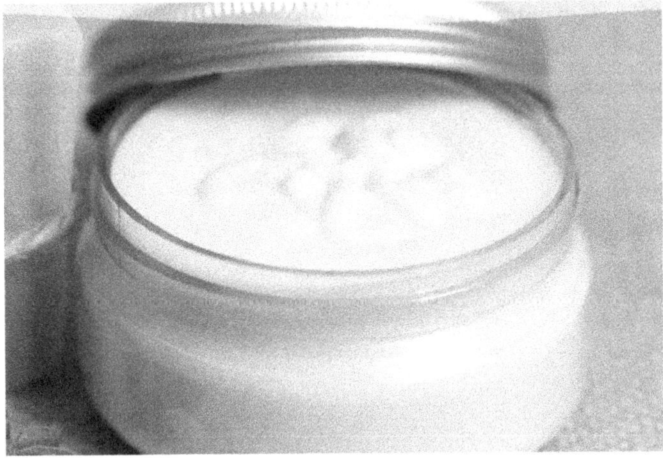

Ingredients:

> ➢ Half cup coconut oil.
> ➢ One tablespoon raw honey.

- ➢ Half cup of shear butter.
- ➢ Five drops of geranium oil.
- ➢ Few drops of lavender essential oil.
- ➢ 7-8 drops of tea tree oil.
- ➢ Five drops of myrrh oil.

Directions:

1. Melt coconut oil and shear butter via a double boiler. (Do not melt them directly on flame).
2. Now pour honey and stir it well.
3. When they are a blend, add both oils and continue to mix them.
4. Cool them till they are semi solid. You can cool them, by putting in the refrigerator for some time. Note: Do not harden mixture.
5. Now you can apply it either in the form of a stand mixer or hand-held. It looks like a bit foamy. Or you can say it resembles lotions.
6. Mix it for every 10 minutes so that it remains a soft liquid.
7. Empty it in Mason jar or any other storage container.
8. You can stock it in the refrigerator or at room temperature. It's better to store it at a room temperature to keep it soft. It will also help to apply easily in a molten form.

22. Dandelion balm Recipe:

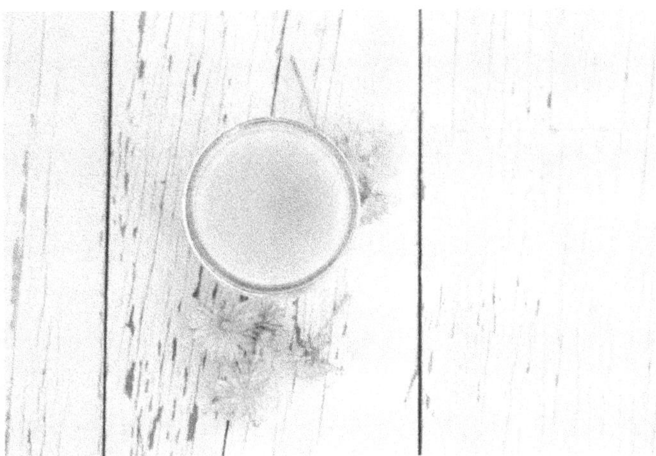

Ingredients:

- ➢ ½ ounce of beeswax pastilles.
- ➢ 3 1/2ounces of dandelion oil.

Directions:

1. Take a heat resistant container and filled it with both ingredients.
2. Place container in a pan containing several inches of water. Boil it in a way that water does not enter into the container.
3. Gently stir, until wax is melted. Alter the temperature from medium to low flame.
4. Remove it from the flame. Empty mixture into jars and let it set for itself. Around 4 ounces of balm will make.

23. Herb- instilled balms:

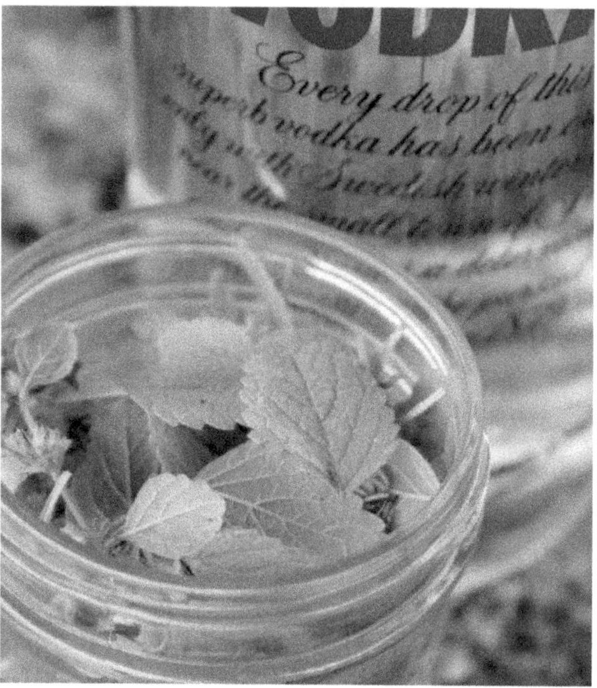

Ingredients:

- ➢ Two tablespoon beeswax.
- ➢ Almond or olive oil.
- ➢ Dried herbs of lavender, calendula and peppermint.
- ➢ Essential oils.
- ➢ Lidded container.

Directions:

1. Preserve oils for 14 to 28 days. In case if fungi grow. Then start this process again.
2. Rinse all the herbs.

3. Take a sauce pan and mix beeswax and oil and heat them up in a double boiler with low flame.
4. Add essential oils when fully melted, then pour in lidded containers.
5. Cool them till they harden. Preserve them in dry and cold place.

24. *Skin healing Balm:*

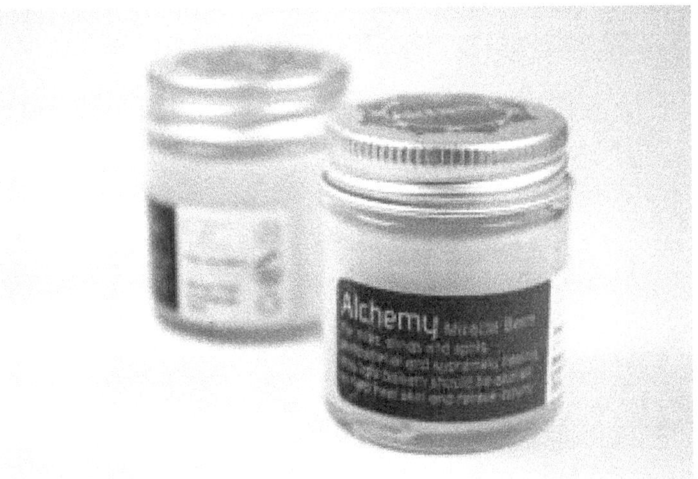

Ingredients:

- ➢ 5 drops of fennel oil.
- ➢ 10 drops of lavender oil.
- ➢ 5 drops of peppermint oil.
- ➢ Few drops of clary sage oil.
- ➢ 1 tablespoon of coconut oil.
- ➢ Equal amount of hemp oil.
- ➢ 1½ tbsp. of grated beeswax.
- ➢ One tbsp. of butter.
- ➢ One tbsp. of almond oil.

Directions:

1. Mix up all ingredients other than essential oils and melt them in double boiler
2. Turn off stove. Add essential oils and mix them.
3. Empty them in pots and let it set by itself.

25. Foot balm:

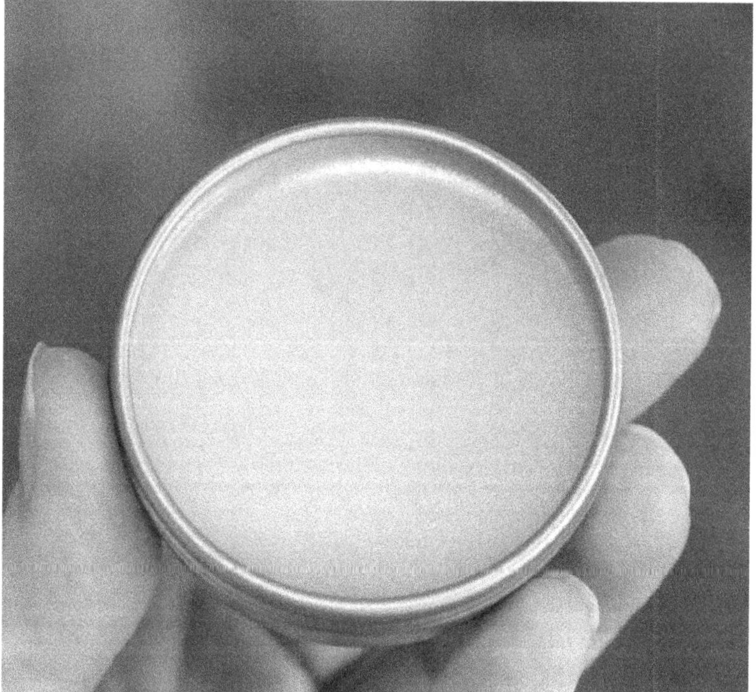

Ingredients:

> Half teaspoon of buckthorn oil.
> Half teaspoon of neem oil.

- ➢ .25 oz of cocoa butter.
- ➢ 4 oz. of lanolin.
- ➢ 1½ oz of olive oil.
- ➢ 1 oz. of beeswax.
- ➢ 1ml rosemary oil.
- ➢ 1ml of lavender oil.
- ➢ 1ml of rosemary extract.
- ➢ .5 oz of shear butter.

Directions:

1. Combine plantain, comfrey, calendula leaves and olive oil in Mason jar.
2. For 4-6 weeks store in dark and cool place.
3. Place Mason jar in pan filled with 2/3 of water. Heat it for 3-4 hours.
4. Let it cool. Now remove excess oil back to jar after passing from cheesecloth.

26. *Plantain herbal balm:*

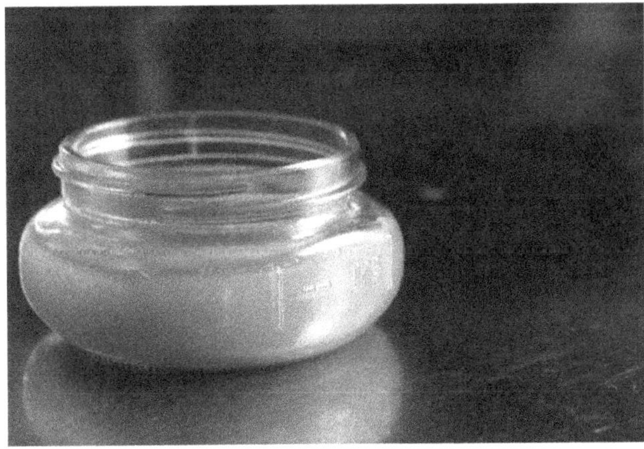

Ingredients:

- ➢ Vitamin E oil.
- ➢ 1 oz beeswax.
- ➢ Grapefruit extract.
- ➢ 4 oz herbal infused oil.

Directions:

1. Mix beeswax and infused oil in a pan. Heat it over low flame with continuous stirring.
2. Once melted, remove from flame.
3. Mix 5 drops of vitamin E oil and grapefruit seed extract.
4. Add other essential oils for fragrance.
5. Add mixture in a porous utensil and let not water mix in it.

27. Natural balm for burn:

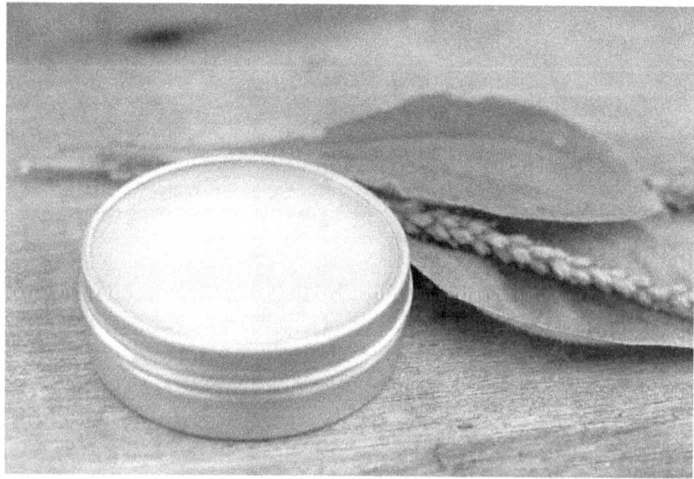

Ingredients:

> ➢ 1 tablespoon Aloe Vera.
> ➢ ¼ cup of honey.
> ➢ 1 tablespoon coconut oil.

Directions:

1. Add all components, mix them and store them in a jar.
2. Prior to its use, apply Apple Cider Vinegar.

28. Boo- boo healing balm:

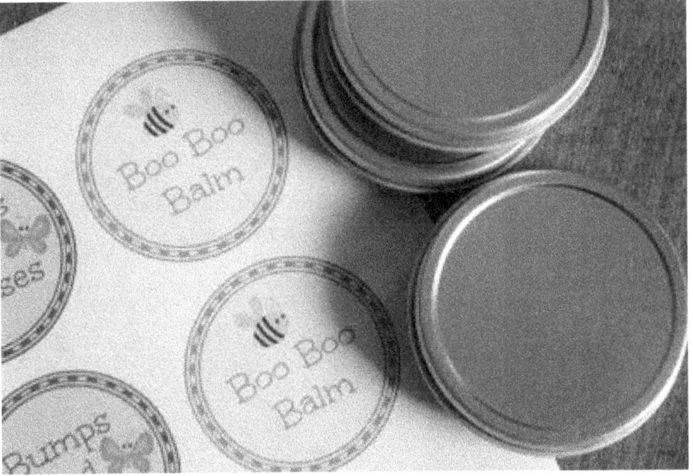

Ingredients:
> ➢ Half cup coconut oil.
> ➢ 1/3 cup dried lavender.
> ➢ Half cup olive oil.
> ➢ 5 drops lavender essential oil.
> ➢ 1/3 cup calendula.
> ➢ 1 tb honey.

- ➢ 10 drops tea tree essential oil.
- ➢ 4 tb beeswax.

Directions:

1. Melt olive and coconut oil in double boiler on low flame.
2. Once melted, add calendula and lavender boil for half hour.
3. Prepare a bowl of coffee filter. Add mixture in it passing from cheese cloth.
4. Again put it on low flame, adding beeswax. After this add honey and cook for 1 minute.
5. Put out flame, add essential oils.
6. Transfer the mixture into jars.

29. Universal balm:

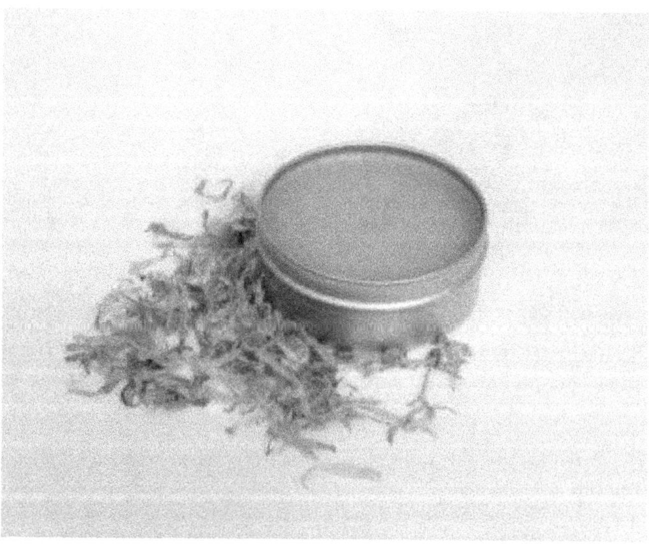

Ingredients:

- ➢ 4 drops of Geranium.

- ➢ 5 drops from tea tree.
- ➢ Half cup of organic jojoba oil.
- ➢ Few drops of lavender oil.
- ➢ Small sprinkle of Vitamin E.
- ➢ ¼ cup of organic almond oil.
- ➢ 2 to 3 spoons of organic neem oil.
- ➢ ¾ tamanu oil.
- ➢ Few drops from Cedar wood.

Directions:

1. Mix all ingredients after measuring.
2. Transfer them into a container.
3. Shake them well.
4. Ready to use.
5. Store in cool and dry place. Shake prior using.

30. Balm for pains in head:

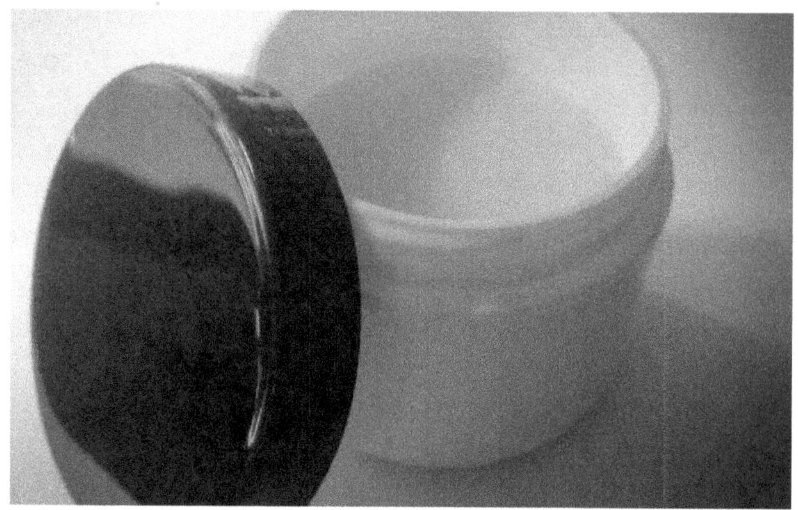

Ingredients:

- 4 tbsp. of olive oil.
- 2tbsp. of shear butter.
- Few drops of peppermint oil.
- 1 oz. of beeswax.
- 20 drops globules oil.
- Drops of Lavender oil.
- 15-20 drops of rosemary oil.
- 1 tbsp. of lemon balm.
- 1 tbsp. of lavender and peppermint leaves each.
- 15 drops of cajuput oil.

Directions:

1. In order to instill oil, take a cloth bag and put herbs in it. Tie it up with a knot so that herbs may not come out of it. (Note: use muslin drawstring bag).
2. Put it in a measuring cup containing enough olive oil in which knotted cloth can easily drown.
3. Transfer cup into a saucepan with a metal ring. You can take ring from canning jar. It will aid cup to settle down at the bottom of pan.
4. Now fill up sauce pan with water in such a way that water reaches to the upper edges of a measuring cup.
5. Heat it until bubble starts forming in water at a medium flame.

Conclusion

The use of herbs and other natural ingredients is not new for treating the injuries and wounds. They have been used for a long time and are proved to be very affecting. This book includes the top recipes for the formation of balms and ointments for healing various kinds of injuries and all of these include the ingredients which are very affective and don't produce any side effect.

A short list of ingredients along with their benefits for health is also included, which is helpful to understand the essential advantages of these remedies. All of the recipes are easy to make and apply while giving the amazing results in less time.

FREE Bonus Reminder

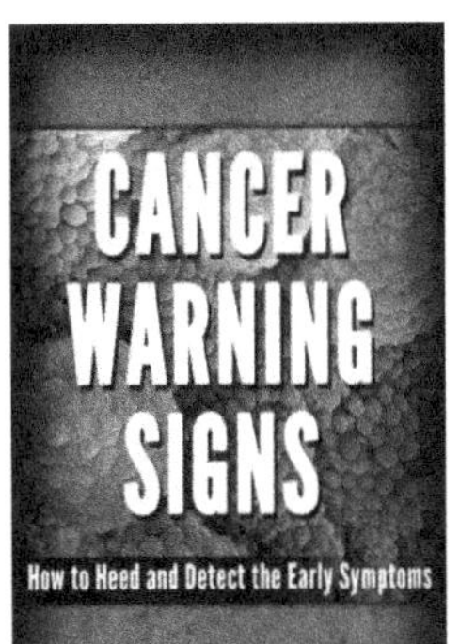

If you have not grabbed it yet, please go ahead and download your special bonus report *"Cancer Warning Signs. How To Heed & Detect The Early Symptoms!"*
Simply Click the Button Below

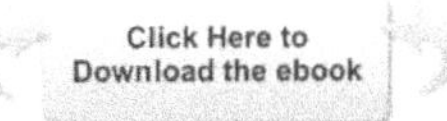

OR **Go to This Page**
http://healthylivingpeople.com/free/

BONUS #2: More Free & Discounted Books or Products
Do you want to receive more Free/Discounted Books or Products?
We have a mailing list where we send out our new Books or Products when they go free or with a discount on Amazon. Click on the link below to sign up for Free & Discount Book & Product Promotions.
=> Sign Up for Free & Discount Book & Product Promotions <=

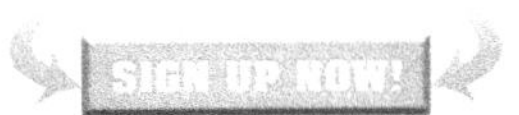

OR Go to this URL
http://zbit.ly/1WBb1Ek